PROSTATE
A Family Affair

PROSTATE
A Family Affair

Harry Elson

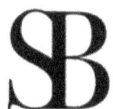

SB

SOFTWOOD BOOKS

SUFFOLK, UK

Throughout this book I have tried to give the most accurate descriptions of medical information, treatments and facilities as I can. Most of the information is already in the public domain.
If, however, there are inaccuracies, I apologise.

If you wish to contact the author about any aspects of this book, please email me at:
noslehm5@gmail.com

Published and manufactured in 2025 by Softwood Books
Reprinted September 2025
EU responsible person: Maddy Glenn
Office 2, Wharfside Road, Prentice Road, Stowmarket, Suffolk, IP14 1RD
www.softwoodbooks.com
hello@softwodbooks.com

EU rep:
Authorised Rep Compliance Ltd., Ground Floor, 71 Lower Baggot Street, Dublin, D02 P593, Ireland
www.arccompliance.com
info@arcompliance.com

ISBN 978-1-83981735-8-6

Dedication
And Thanks

My heartfelt thanks to the unwavering support of Clare and Sarah at the Royal Surrey Oncology Department.

To my wife, Margaret (M), who has trod this path with me and lived every moment, being my taxi driver, drug administrator and editor.

To Jeremy, Tim and David who have shared their cancer battles with me.

To Simon: good choice of Palatino typeface!

To Catriona for scrutinising the manuscript with her "fine-toothed comb".

To Softwood Books and the team – many thanks – again.

**the
PROSTATE
project**

giving men a better chance
of beating prostate cancer

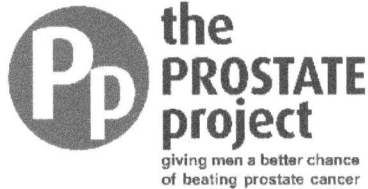

All profits from sales of this book will be donated to the Prostate Project – a cancer charity which is dedicated to raising awareness and funds to help save and prolong the lives of men with prostate cancer.

Based at the Royal Surrey County Hospital in Guildford, and run almost entirely by volunteers, in the 25 years since its foundation the Prostate Project has raised over £8million.

www.prostate-project.org.uk

Thank you for your purchase of this book.

Contents

Introduction

I had always been the "Elephant in the Room": encouraging my peers to get checked – a simple PSA test is a start. I would say that most of them were unaware of what is a PSA test.

What is PSA?

Prostate-Specific Antigen is a protein produced by the prostate gland and a PSA test is a simple blood test that measures the amount of PSA. The test is used to detect problems, such as prostate infection, enlarged prostate, and cancer, all of which can then be investigated. You may have heard, or been told, that the test is not accurate and it is true that it can vary from man to man, but having an annual test will give you a benchmark to make comparisons.

Who should get a PSA test? Men aged 50 or over, men of any age with a family history of prostate cancer and men of any age who are experiencing pain in the prostate area or pain when peeing and, of course, the need to get up in the night to pee.

What are the risks and benefits of a PSA test? There are no risks, apart from a few days of worry if a high reading is shown,. Even if this is the case, please bear in mind that false positive results can happen occasionally. The benefits do, however, speak for themselves; any problem with the prostate can then be further investigated with MRI, CT scans or biopsy.

How to get a PSA test
The NHS does not offer routine testing, but a visit to your GP should enable this procedure. You may have a battle with the GP to get this, but do persevere if you are concerned.

PSA levels and age
Normal PSA levels can vary from man to man but, generally, levels increase with age.

What is a high PSA level?
A tricky question to answer as levels do vary from individual to individual. But, generally speaking, according to Cancer Research UK:

Below 4.0 – 15% chance of cancer
Between 4.0 and 10.0 (borderline range) – 25% chance of cancer
Above 10.0 – greater than 50% chance of cancer.

INTRODUCTION

I was proud that, for many years, I had religiously had an annual PSA and blood test, so felt confident that I would not follow my father down the dark road of prostate cancer. But I did.

This silent killer had been waiting for me: could I have done anything more – yes or no?

We all rely on our GPs' expertise, but they are only human and one can, therefore, question their knowledge and diagnosis. Even as I write, in June 2025, there still appears to be a reluctance on the part of some GPs to investigate anything that may be linked to prostate problems. It still has the stigma of the "old man's disease".

Prostate cancer is now the most common cancer in men in the UK. The prostate is a small gland in the pelvis and is part of the male reproductive system. It is located below the bladder and just in front of the back passage (rectum). Urine from the bladder passes through the centre of the prostate and along the water pipe (urethra) to leave the body at the end of the penis.

The primary function of the prostate gland is to produce and secrete fluid that contributes to semen. This prostatic fluid, rich in enzymes and other substances, nourishes and protects sperm. aiding in their motility and viability. Additionally, the prostate's muscular contractions play a role in the ejaculation process, helping to propel semen out of the body. When cancer is found early, and confined to the prostate, it often shows no symptoms and can only be detected by testing.

I decided to write this book as it seemed to me that there was such a "Russian Roulette" approach to detection of prostate cancer. I felt that if I could save just one man, it would be well worth putting pen to paper.

You may wonder why there are the "male and female" symbols on the cover of this book. The reason for this is that is it increasingly being shown that there is a link between prostate and ovarian cancers.

My own sister died of ovarian cancer without it being detected until it was too late. One of my maternal aunts also suffered with it, but, fortunately, hers was caught in its early stages and proved treatable.

WANTED!

PROSTATE: THE SILENT KILLER

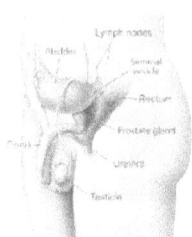

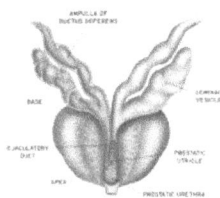

A small gland located below the bladder

IT MAY BE SMALL, BUT IT'S DEADLY

FACTS:

More than 12,000 deaths in the UK each year.

More than 55,000 new cases in the UK each year.

Get your PSA checked!

See your GP if you have any symptoms.

Don't let your GP brush you off; he or she might not have the knowledge.

ACT NOW!

Chapter One
INTO THE UNKNOWN

I became aware of prostate cancer in my forties and made sure to always have blood tests when undertaking my annual check-ups with BUPA. In 2002, when I was 56, my PSA was 0.8 (low).

As the years went by, I was often thinking about my father's death, in 1990, from prostate cancer, so thought I would go and see my GP to discuss whether there was any possibility of inheriting the disease. He agreed that I should have annual PSA tests, together with digital rectal examinations if he felt the situation required it, but he would advise accordingly. I felt reassured.

When I was 64 my 2010 test showed a reading of 1.0 – a small rise, but my GP wasn't concerned, stating that such a rise was "quite normal" for my age.

In 2019, I was 73, my annual PSA test reading showed a considerable rise to 2.6, so my GP carried out a digital rectal examination after which he said he considered that my prostate was slightly enlarged and felt "rough" on the left side. But, he assured me, no action was necessary – *wrong!*

Hindsight is always a wonderful thing and, I often wonder, if only I had done this or that, would the outcome have been different.

My everlasting regret is that I had complete faith in my GP. I am, however, thankful that my own experience has urged others, including my son, to get tested and, where required, treatment.

Chapter Two
FAMILY HISTORY

D ad's gradual decline was clear for all to see. He was 80 years old when he died in 1990 and had been a very fit man up until he was 75, working full-time as a gardener for all of his life. He had been a superb sportsman in his younger days: both cricket and football featured large in his life.

I can't remember exactly when, but he suffered a slight fall and began to complain about a pain in his hip, but put it down to wear and tear. He saw his GP who said it was just that – *wrong!*

In fairness to his GP, this was a time when prostate cancer wasn't really talked about; it was still the "old man's disease" and I am sure it didn't even occur to him to consider what it might be. Indeed, my father had never heard of prostate cancer and he had no idea what it might do to his body.

As the years went on, Dad started to limp and began using a stick, becoming increasingly less mobile. Then, one evening, my mother rang to say that Dad had collapsed. He was admitted to the old St. Luke's Hospital in Warren Road, Guildford. In the first week he did have some radiotherapy treatment, but died within two weeks. The prostate cancer had spread silently over the years to his bones, then when his pelvis failed, he collapsed. He was never to walk again.

Following this episode I thought I would never let myself face this end – *wrong!*

But, thankfully, it isn't "the end". I am, however, facing my own prostate cancer battle.

Interestingly, Dad had two brothers who both died of prostate cancer. Could it be that my family carried a faulty gene?

Then there was my sister, who was fit and well for her entire life, but often complained about a pain in her lower left side which seemed to also affect her leg. She didn't ever seek medical advice and just put up with it (that's the "Elson" way). During a trip to Canada she fell sick and on her return to the UK she was diagnosed with ovarian cancer. She had surgery to remove the cancerous ovaries, and this seemed to be successful, being followed up with a course of chemotherapy. Within months, however, the aggressive cancer had returned with a vengeance and she died soon after.

One of my maternal aunts was also diagnosed with ovarian cancer but in her case it was caught early on and she recovered – she is still alive today. My maternal grandmother and several other aunts also suffered from various forms of cancer.

A shock was to come: my son when my son, Jeremy, then aged 57, was diagnosed with early prostate cancer later in 2022. (Please read his account in Personal Accounts, page 69).

We shall see later how The Royal Marsden Hospital (Chapter Eleven) investigated the family genome and what their findings were into the genetic pointers of this deadly disease.

Chapter Three
ONE YEAR ON

I n 2020 I had my annual blood test and follow-up with my GP – my PSA reading had risen to 3.7 (2.6 the previous year). This, he advised me, was within the age-related PSA references for caucasian men, so I felt reassured as he also carried out another digital rectal examination and continued to assure me that there was nothing abnormal – *wrong!*

At this meeting I told him that I had been feeling a sensation in my groin area, but he said this was nothing to be concerned about and would not be linked to my prostate

Over the next 10 months I had no real symptoms that could be linked to any prostate problem. But, with the benefit of hindsight, and my family history, I should have pushed him for further tests and investigation.

Then, in October 2021, during one of my visits to Spain, I began to experience a very uncomfortable feeling in my prostate area and also began waking up at night – the alarm bells started ringing.

On my return to the UK in late November 2021, I immediately contacted my GP for my annual PSA test. Soon after the test, I was contacted by the surgery to make an appointment for a follow-up.

As luck would have it, my usual GP was not available and I was seen by a different GP who seemed to have significantly more knowledge about prostate issues, explaining that my latest reading had now risen to 7.69 (previously 3.7 – it had doubled in a year) and that he had referred me for further investigation. The doctor was concerned, especially given my family history, which he took very seriously. This needed, he said, immediate action at the hospital.

There followed the start of my many investigations at the St Luke's Cancer Centre at the RSCH (Royal Surrey County Hospital) in Guildford. It has just this year been renamed the Royal Surrey Cancer Centre.

Chapter Four
INVESTIGATIONS

I attended the Oncology Department at the Royal Surrey County Hospital (RSCH) for an MRI scan on the 13th January 2022 – all very quick and professional.

Magnetic Resonance Imaging (MRI) scanning uses strong magnetic fields and radio waves to create detailed images of the inside of the body. It is quick, easy and painless; all you need to do is lie still inside the MRI scanner for about 25 minutes. It is a little disconcerting as there are continual loud clicking and whirring sounds. Earplugs are usually supplied, but you are still aware of all the noises!

With the results still pending, I was surprised to be immediately referred for a biopsy on my prostate. I didn't know what to expect.

Should I look it up online to find out what it was all about? – I didn't!

On the fateful day, the 17th January 2022, I again attended the St Luke's Cancer Centre. I arrived at the normal waiting area, booked in and entered the room, still not knowing what to expect. At first, I thought I was in the wrong room – in front of me was a chair with leg supports, such as you see in a maternity delivery room!

I had to sit in the chair with my legs apart and raised in the supports (as if ready to give birth!). There was much reassurance of what was to come. A very nice member of staff held my hand and gave words of support and comfort as I was administered a local anaesthetic – all very reassuring.

I had a probe inserted into my anus to aid the process of the biopsy. Then the first "shot" as I call it as they take tissue from the prostate. Sixteen "shots" in all! It was uncomfortable and I was given plenty of reassurances throughout. Overall, in hindsight, it wasn't too bad.

My son, Jeremy, also had to experience this same procedure and it has become the subject of our black humour, causing many hilarious exchanges. (See his story in Personal Accounts, page 69, where he goes into plenty of detail!).

The report to my GP following the biopsy stated:

"I saw Mr Harold Elson in the Urology Fast Track Prostate Clinic recently. This gentleman was referred to us due to a slightly elevated PSA of 7.65.

Mr Elson has a positive family history of prostatic adenocarcinoma which affected his father. A multiparametric MRI scan was performed which showed a prostate size of 75ml alongside the left-sided suspicious area which was affecting the left hemigland with a possible extracapsular extension of PI-RADS 5. There were also positive bilateral pelvic lymph nodes and suspicious left posterior acetabular osseous disease.

A digital rectal examination carried out revealed a hard prostate affecting the left lobe. I explained all these findings to Mr Elson and that a prostate biopsy was recommended.

Mr Elson agreed to undergo a transperineal prostate biopsy under local anaesthetic which I performed for him after explaining the full details of the procedure, along with possible side effects and complications.

Mr Elson was given a pre-operative Ciprofloxacin 500mg to reduce the chance of infection. Multiple four quadrant biopsies were taken and he tolerated the procedure very well under a local anaesthetic. He was kept under observation in the waiting area for a period of time and then discharged home.

I explained to Mr Elson of the need to return to the hospital should he develop any complications or side effects after the procedure and we will be happy to see him through the emergency channels. We will be in touch again in due course regarding the outcome of the prostate biopsy and the need for further treatment and/or investigations if required."

[Senior Robotic Fellow]

What are PI-RADS?

PI-RADS stands for Prostate Imaging Reporting and Data System. On a scale of 1 to 5, a reading of 1 means most likely not cancer and 5 means very suspicious.

On the 25th January the Urology Department wrote to the Oncology Department:

"I would be very grateful if you could review this 75-year old man who has a family history of prostate cancer. His father died, aged 80, from metastatic prostate cancer. Mr Elson has monitored his PSA for some years and it was within the normal range in 2019. He was referred with a PSA of 7.6 under the two week rule guidelines.

An MRI showed PI-RADS 5 disease affecting the whole left side of his prostate with likely lymph node involvement and an abnormal area of the left acetabulum indicating a possible bone met. His biopsies have shown left sided disease Gleason 5+5=10 with a maximum tumour focus of 12 cores and 6 cores from the left anterior and 5+4=9 in 5 cores from the left posterior.

[See the next page for a description of the Gleason score]

I have informed Mr Elson of the results and explained the MRI results to him along with our suspicion of metastatic disease. I have requested a bone scan and a CT scan, and I am very grateful to you for reviewing him when these scans are available. He is aware that his first line of treatment will be hormones followed by likely some form of chemotherapy.

He is very fit and well and is not on any regular medication. He has no allergies and very little in the way of lower urinary tract symptoms.

He has a house in Spain and was hoping to travel there for four or five weeks at the end of February. I have advised him that, although a short trip to Spain is not out of the question, to travel there for four or five weeks, particularly if he requires chemotherapy may not be advisable at this stage. He is willing to change his travel arrangements but will wait until he has had his appointment with you and the result of the scans.

I am very grateful to you for reviewing him.

[Prostate Cancer Clinical Nurse Specialist]

Gleason Score

One important component of staging cancer is its grade. Traditionally, prostate cancer grades are described according to the Gleason Score, a system named after the pathologist, Dr Donald Gleason, who developed it in the 1960s, when he realised that cancerous cells fall into five distinct patterns as they change from normal cells to tumour cells. Cells are graded on a scale of 1 to 5. Grade 1 cells resemble normal prostate tissue whilst those closest to 5 are considered "high grade" and have mutated so much that they barely resemble normal cells.

The pathologist will assign one Gleason Grade to the most predominant pattern in the sample and a second Gleason Grade to the second most dominant, pattern. For example: 3+4, the two grades will be added together to determine the Gleason Score.

A Gleason Score of 6 is low grade, 7 is intermediate and 8 to 10 is high grade. Theoretically, Gleason scores range from 2-10 but below 5 is almost never assigned now.

The next meeting was with was the Consultant Clinical Oncologist on the 4th February 2002. He outlined the contents of the letters that had been sent to him by the Urology Department and said that we would need to start treatment immediately. This would take the form of Zoladex injections and, to my surprise, he carried out the first procedure there and then.

Zoladex is an implant injection used as a hormone therapy which prevents the testicles from producing testosterone, thereby lowering testosterone levels from which the cancer feeds itself.

He wrote to my GP on the 4th February 2002 with the diagnosis stating:

I have spoken to Mr Elson today. He had a CT chest, abdomen and pelvis and a bone scan in February 2022. Those confirmed metastatic disease affecting the cervical spine, sternum and left acetabulum. CT chest, abdomen and pelvis showed retroperitoneal lymphadenopathy, pelvic lymph nodes.

He will need to continue with the LHRH analogues long-term. I will administer the next monthly injection today but you will need to organise a three-monthly Zoladex injection of 10.8mg for the first week of April 2022.

[LHRH stands for Left Hemigland and Right Hemigland; i.e. One half of the prostate gland]

Mr Elson has consented to systemic chemotherapy with Docetaxel which is a Cytotoxic taxane agent with an aim to downstage the disease, prolong life expectancy, improve outcomes. Potential side effects of chemotherapy include the risk of neutopenic sepsis, thromboembolic disease, fatigue, nausea.

Mr Elson has consented for chemotherapy with Docetaxel and we will see him in clinic for treatment.

[Consultant Clinical Oncologist]

During the meeting my Consultant was very interested in my family history as he said that there was a good chance I had inherited a faulty gene from my father. He suggested that he contact The Royal Marsden Hospital to arrange an appointment to investigate the matter further. The letter read:

"I would grateful if you would organise BRCA testing for this 75-year old patient. His sister passed away with ovarian cancer several years ago. His father was

22

diagnosed with prostate cancer, now he himself has been diagnosed with aggressive prostate cancer. This raises the likelihood of a germline BRCA mutation. Even though, currently, he is not within the national guidance, in his case, in view of the family history, BRCA testing is considered necessary and may change his management."

I did proceed and visited The Royal Marsden Hospital in Sutton for genetic profiling which is covered later in the book (Chapter Eleven).

What is BRCA?

BRCA stands for BReast CAncer. Everyone has BRCA1 and BRCA2 genes. They are important genes that stop the cells in our body from growing and dividing out of control. Doctors call these the tumour suppressor genes.

A gene change in BRCA1 or BRCA2 means that the cells can grow out of control which can lead to the development of cancer. A change to BRCA1 and BRCA2 is rare. Only around one in every 400 people have a change in both genes.

Ethnicity can also affect the risk of carrying gene changes. Both men and women can have a change in BRCA1 or BRCA2. People who inherit versions of these changed genes have an increased risk of developing different types of cancers. People with a BRCA mutation may be up to six times more likely to develop cancers. These include, breast cancer, ovarian cancer, prostate cancer and pancreatic cancer.

I had another MRI scan on the 6th February 2022 and on the 10th a bone scan – this is very different as it uses a radioactive substance which is injected into the blood stream. You have to wait for four hours after the injection of the substance and then the scan is carried out.

Waiting for the results was a difficult time as inevitably one always thinks the worst. That day came on the 4th March 2022, a week before my 76th birthday and will go down as a low point in my life.

Why? Because I had done just about everything possible to make sure that I would not be struck down with this silent killer as my father had been.

Ten years of PSA testing and examinations, only to be let down – and this is my own opinion – by a GP who should have taken notice of my family history and sent me for a thorough check-up a year before when my PSA had doubled. There could have been a very different outcome to my treatment. One continually reads about the importance of early testing and diagnosis but it seems that some GPs are still not acting on this.

On the 18th March 2022, Margaret came with me for support as we went to the Oncology Department to hear the outcome of all the tests and discuss the way forward, including procedures for the forthcoming chemotherapy treatment.

The only good news at this meeting was that due to the Zoladex hormone implant, my PSA had dropped to 2.5. The die was cast, however, for my next few months when I would have chemotherapy every three weeks for six sessions.

I cannot express how angry and disappointed I was at the news. It was devastating: I felt that I had done everything possible not to be in this situation – but here I was with prostate cancer of the worst form: Stage Four.

I was told that there would, initially, be a course of six sessions of chemotherapy, one every three weeks and I would be continuing with the three-monthly injections of Zoladex – forever, it seems!

Chapter Five
CHEMOTHERAPY

My chemotherapy treatment began on the 23rd March 2022. This was at the Chilworth Ward oft The Royal Surrey Cancer Centre (still known as St Luke's at this time).

Coincidentally, Jeremy, one of my sons, was at the same hospital having a scan in relation to his own prostate screening which had been recommended by his GP due to the family history. (See his story in Personal Accounts, page 69)

There were lots of thoughts going through my head as I turned up at St Luke's for my first treatment.

I had never spoken to anyone about the procedure and was not sure exactly what to expect. I turned up at Reception and went through a booking-in process, was given a number and made my way to a room where there were approximately 10 large chairs arranged around the sides of the room.

It was all very busy and professional. I sat down and was seen by a nurse who went through my details and gave me a wristband with barcodes and information. The next step: another nurse inserted a cannula into my arm, ready to take the chemotherapy solution via a drip.

Another nurse came up with a mobile stand and the pouch with the chemotherapy liquid was attached. I was hooked up and the slow-drip process started. My first dose lasted about an hour. I sat there and whiled away the time by reading or looking at my i-Pad, not really talking to anyone. Everyone seemed to be in their own world, the same as me. I saw a noticeboard on the wall showing patients' names and types of chemotherapy they were being given. It seemed to me that each patient received a unique prescription.

As an aside, the coffee and biscuits, soup, sandwiches and fruit were very enjoyable. During the Wimbledon Tennis Tournament we were served strawberries and cream by wonderful ladies dressed as strawberries! What a lovely lift to our flagging spirits that was! Thank you, lovely ladies!

My own prescription was for Docetaxel which is a chemotherapy drug used to treat various cancers, including prostate cancer. It is a taxane, a type of chemotherapy which disrupts microtubules, cellular structures that help chromosomes move during cell division. By inactivating microtubule bundles, Docetaxel stops mitosis (a type of cell division that results in two genetically identical daughter cells from a single parent cell) and prevents cancer cells from growing and spreading.

The day before my treatment, I had been told to take a Dexamethazone tablet, a corticosteroid medication that treats inflammation and reduces the body's immune response – basically, an anti-sickness treatment – and also Bicalututamide, a non-steroidal, oral hormone therapy tablet used in the treatment of prostate cancer which prevents testosterone from reaching cancer cells on the day.

Worse was to come: three days after each treatment I had to administer an injection of Nivestim, a medicine that stimulates the production of white blood cells in the bone marrow. This was to help my body be more able to fight infection. The injections had to be administered daily for five days and given in the front or side of my thighs.

It was a bit disconcerting the first time that Margaret and I did this but, gradually, one gets used to the process and it becomes a matter of routine, as everything does eventually.

Chemotherapy is always a leap into the unknown and my second cycle which commenced in August 2025 brought on a dramatic chain of events. I have documented these in Chapter 10, "Looking to the Future".

Chapter Six
AND THEN WHAT?

I was obviously aware of the likely side effects having read the literature provided by the hospital describing the possibilities – but this was a huge list!

When you realise that the chemotherapy drug effectively kills off both good and bad cells and actually poisons your system, it is not surprising that there are side effects.

I had no immediate problems, but gradually I had the common symptoms: my hair was starting to thin and then my body hair disappeared altogether. My shaving habits changed due to this slowing down of hair growth. My finger and toe nails began to be affected – they became very dry and ridged. Later into the treatment, the nerves in my feet and lower legs were affected by neuropathy (nerve damage) – a strange, tingling peripheral feeling which I still have to this day.

AND THEN WHAT?

The consequence of chemotherapy affecting one's immune system is very serious. I only experienced this once: two months into my treatment. It was the worst experience I had ever encountered and I was knocked sideways, unable to stand and completely lost control of my bodily functions. I only started to recover after two days. It was a terrible time.

I had always had a very positive attitude to my treatment. Prior to my diagnosis, I was very fit for my age and now I continued with my normal routine: keeping up my exercise regime on my static bike, eating well, treating myself to my usual daily beer, and so forth.

I was lucky to have a property in Spain and visited between treatments – the sun always made me feel better.

I had monthly review meetings with the Clinical Oncology Department at the St Luke's Cancer Centre. These could be face-to-face or over the phone. At these meetings I was given feedback on my PSA, which at this time was going down.

I felt that my body was changing noticeably and my muscle strength was diminishing, but I cover that in more detail in the next chapter.

Chapter Seven
HORMONE
TREATMENT

I survived the chemotherapy treatment and, to my surprise, apart from the incident noted earlier, did not feel sick or ill. In fact, I seemed to be back to my normal self, except for the ongoing neuropathy which caused me problems – overall, a small cost to pay.

I think that far worse is the ongoing hormone treatment which continues to this day and probably will do so for the rest of my life. It has affected me badly and in different ways to the chemotherapy.

Zoladex is a type of hormone therapy used to treat metastatic and locally-advanced prostate cancer through the suppression of testosterone and is administered at three monthly intervals via a spring-loaded implant injection. It works by reducing levels of sex hormones (testosterone) in the body, resulting in the reduction of PSA levels.

And then, and then... my body started to really change: I never had any fat around my tummy area but this has changed dramatically now. I do not eat any more than I did before (actually less, I think) and I still cannot believe that I have a belly! Of all the things, I really hate what these drugs are doing to my body.

And, without going into too much detail my sexual equipment has also changed and my sex drive is now zero. Another monumental change in my life.

Another strange phenomenon is that when I am working in the garden, I have to stop just as if I suddenly have zero energy and the tap has been turned off. I now have to sit down to recover (my wife says it's also my age, I am not 21 any more! but I know the drugs are a contributory factor).

A consequence of spending five or six weeks in Spain is that I have to make arrangements for my Zoladex implant while I am there. I take my implant "injection" with me (I can get it through security at Gatwick!). The process is actually very easy: the local private hospital has an excellent booking-in system: you tap in at a screen terminal and select the option you want (out-patients) and get a ticket printed out. When your number appears on the screen you go to one of the fifteen booking-in desks, provide your details and what you require. Pay the 15 Euros and go to an "out-patients" area. Wait for your number to be called – go into a treatment room: lift your shirt up, implant administered.

Off you go.

No laying on a couch with several sheets of paper which are discarded immediately afterwards. Excellent use of resources, minimal waste – a good result all round.

I know one shouldn't compare, but here in the UK, I have to book in for my appointment with the nurse six weeks before I need my implant to be administered. I realise that I pay 15 Euros in Spain but I just turn up on the day – job done.

Chapter Eight
ONGOING REVIEWS

In October 2022 I had repeated scans (CT, MRI and Bone). This was to see just how effective the chemotherapy had been.

The response was very positive in that the cancer that had been identified from my first scans had significantly reduced. As I stated earlier, after the chemotherapy I noticed I was affected by neuropathy which resulted in a strange (and very unpleasant) tingling sensation in my feet an legs.

I also had periods of listlessness and feeling drained but kept up my fitness routine as much as I could – dancing with M, static bike, lifting weights and using my punchball.

By November, I was feeling much better – my hair was starting to return and thicken and my nails were improving. Unfortunately, the neuropathy was here to stay and has been the main side effect of the treatment and it is still with me every night when it is at its worst. Having always been a sound sleeper, I now regularly wake two, or even, three times every night: a short walk round, a quick drink or a quick pee and I go back to bed. It is not good and I am sure that this is a contributing factor to the tiredness that I feel during the day. M always used to wake up when I went "walk-about" but now, it seems, she sleeps through it.

I continued with regular blood tests, Zoladex implants and meetings. My PSA reading had gone from 7.6 to 0.372 as of the 11th April 2023.

I also continued to have CT, Bone and MRI scans at regular intervals and on the 21st July 2023 my PSA stood at 0.42 – it was starting to rise. Not a good sign, I thought. It was, therefore, decided that I should have a PET scan.

PET stands for Positron Emission Tomography and is a medical imaging technique that uses radioactive tracers to visualise and measure changes in metabolic processes and physiological activities within the body. A radioactive iodine is injected into the blood stream. Another painless and relatively quick procedure.

By the 15th September my PSA had again risen to 0.7 – time for action. The Oncology Team were concerned at this rise, and felt that it was a sign that my current treatment was losing effectiveness. The recommendation was to administer Abiraterone, a prescription-based drug, used to treat advanced prostate cancer in men, as a safeguard.

Abiraterone is a type of hormone therapy for men with prostate cancer that has spread to other parts of the body (advanced prostate cancer). It works by preventing the production of testosterone. It does this in a different way than other types of hormone therapy. In most men, prostate cancer cells can't grow without testosterone, even if the cancer has spread to other parts of the body. Abiraterone doesn't cure prostate cancer, but it can help keep it under control and has been shown to help some men live longer. It can also help to treat or delay symptoms, such as pain and tiredness.

NHS England now funds Abariterone in line with NICE's recommendations, making it routinely available for the treatment of advanced prostate cancer. It is an expensive drug, costing in the region of £2,930 for 120 tablets (in my case 60 days' supply).

Abiraterone is usually used in conjunction with Prednisolone, a corticosteroid medication that treats a variety of inflammatory, hormonal and auto-immune conditions.

My current dosage is two tablets (500gm) of Abiraterone each morning before food, taken with my morning cuppa and two biscuits!. I also take two tablets of Prednisolone (5mg) one with breakfast, the other with lunch.

The administration of Abiraterone was successful and by November 2023 my PSA reading had, once again, reduced to 0.16.

These treatments have, however, seemed to exacerbated the effects of Zoladex and there has now been an added problem to my interrupted sleep. I also suffer from bruising at the slightest knock to my arms and legs – a terrible drawback to someone who is used to working in the garden, cleaning cars etc.

Recently, I was doing some work in the garden and gashed one of my arms – not too bad, but we decided to put a bandage over it with a couple of plasters. The plasters bruised my skin and it took several weeks for the bruises to disappear.

Three-monthly reviews continued throughout the next year with blood tests for PSA readings, but in November 2024 my PSA was starting to rise again. I then went through the procedure of scans: CT, Bone and PET.

At my review on the 20th December 2024, the feedback was better than expected: none of the scans showed any evidence of cancer. It was, therefore, recommended that the same treatment be continued (Abiraterone and Zoladex) but more investigation would be needed as to why my PSA was on the rise.

My April 2025 review showed that my PSA had, once again, risen – now 3.1 (still not a lot) and nothing to be concerned about yet. My oncologist advised that she would be more concerned if the reading was "leaping" rather than "creeping" up.

The next step in three months time (July) after the usual blood tests could be more scans and the possibility of different treatment and/or chemotherapy – not something I look forward to.

These are always booked via a letter from the Oncology Department who advise the next review date. It is not app driven but paper driven, so I have to book myself in for a specific blood test. Once my blood is diagnosed the next step is determined. Even the blood tests are not simple: once booked via the on-line site, I have to advise a member of the Oncology team of my appointment so they can get me booked into the "system".

There appears to be no joined up thinking whatsoever but, as I have found, the people I deal with are very helpful.

My Treatment Regime, three years on:

Daily	2 x Abiraterone, before food
Daily	2 x Predinisolone (one with breakfast, one with lunch)
Three monthly	Zoladedx implant
Three monthly	Blood test for PSA and then follow-up with Oncologist. Booked via the app and a visit to the Phebolotomy department at RSCH. This is reviewed and any changes to my PSA can be referred for further investigation and/or treatment

---

Zoladex and Abiraterone
My partners in crime.
I thought you deserved a poetical line.

ZOLADEX

Oh, Zoladex, how wonderful to know,
Every three months, in you go!
Do I feel better for your ingress?
Another three years and I'll be wearing
a dress!

ABIRATERONE

Abiraterone, you sound so strange.
An answer to all my dreams?
Two tablets daily I have to take,
Forever, now it seems.

Chapter Nine
ADDED STRESS

Having to travel to St Luke's Cancer Unit by car, I was fortunate enough to be dropped off by Margaret (M) as we live within two miles of the centre.

Always battling the traffic and the everyday problems that come with driving, on arriving at the centre, the lack of parking facilities becomes immediately apparent. We were provided with a car park pass, but there were never any spaces.

I always felt very sorry for those people who had travelled many miles to see their consultant or for on-going tests and treatments that can go on indefinitely. Parking problems just add to the stress.

You just do not realise, until you are confronted with the problem, the number of times you have to turn up for different meetings, scans, tests, medication collections, etc. Prior to the review, one always has to have a blood test for PSA, so there are always at least two visits for each review meeting. And then at least another visit to collect the drugs from the hospital pharmacy.

A number of my friends who have had radiotherapy had to visit these places on a daily basis, often for several weeks. Travelling to and from the hospital is already stressful, without the added hassle of finding a parking space, especially when you are on the clock.

I don't know what the answer is, but let's hope that there may be one on the horizon.

I just don't know how people who rely on public transport manage such visits – maybe I am not aware of an alternative, although I believe that there is a transport scheme in place, if required. I have had many conversations with people in the car park who have started their journey at an ungodly hour only to find there is nowhere to park.

Chapter Ten
LOOKING TO THE FUTURE?

S o, here we are, still riding the wave of optimism.

I am now in my 79th year, still taking the tablets and visiting St Luke's Cancer Centre on a regular basis.

I am still in good health, enjoying my visits to Spain and keeping myself active. I am always encouraged to read in the press about the breakthroughs being made on new treatments to combat prostate cancer. Unfortunately, they always seem so far off. I am also concerned that the Government of the day still has not come up with a national screening plan as I feel that so many men are missing the chance for early treatment. My own experience has shown that the GP system is not always effective.

It depresses me that I meet so many men, young men of a certain age, who are completely oblivious to this killer disease or, even if they aware of it, think it won't happen to them.

It is, however, encouraging to note that with a number of high-profile personalities succumbing to this disease, there has been a lot of press and media coverage. One hopes that this will kick-start the Government into commencing a screening programme such as is available for women in the form of breast and cervical cancers.

I have written this as a window into my own experience. These are my views and I would not wish anyone to think that I was being negative – on the contrary, since my diagnosis, my view on the treatments I have received has been wholly positive.

I would like to add that if you are reading this book and are suffering from a prostate problem, please remain positive because there is still much life after the diagnosis.

And then the Curved Ball arrived
In August 2025, I began my second cycle of chemotherapy. It was a variation from the previous

one but I was assured that it was tailored to my needs.

A few days later I developed neutropenic sepsis and was admitted to hospital. It took more than three days to start to recover and a further seven days to get back to fitness.

I now realise just how serious this condition is but am glad to say I have fully recovered.

My thanks to the paramedic team from the Surrey Ambulance Service and the medics at the Frimley Park Hospital whose prompt action helped me to survive.

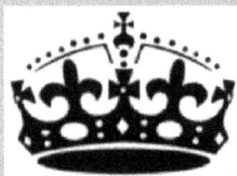

KEEP CALM

AND

BOOK A

PSA

TEST

CARRY ON, DON'T DELAY

Chapter Eleven
THE ROYAL
MARSDEN HOSPITAL

Following my meeting with the Consultant Clinical Oncologist at St Luke's Cancer Centre, I was contacted by the Royal Marsden with information about Prostate Cancer Genetic Research Studies. The Oncologenetics Research Team informed me that I could take part in:

The Precision Medicine in the Prostate Cancer Care Pathway: an evaluation of integrating germline genetic testing into the management of men at risk of/living with prostate cancer.

The Purpose of the Study:
Men with a certain genetic make-up may be more likely to develop prostate cancer. We are inviting men who either have prostate cancer, or who are closely related to

someone with prostate cancer, to have research genetic testing. The genetic test will analyse a sample of our DNA (genetic material) for a set of genes that are known to be important in the development of prostate cancer and how this might inform clinical management.

We will look at how genetic information may be used to guide the types of treatments that men with prostate cancer can be offered both now and in the future. We will also look at different screening options for men who are found to have a genetic predisposition, but who have not yet developed prostate cancer.

Cancer is generally caused by a combination of many factors, and research tells us that the main things that increase your risk of getting prostate cancer are age, having a family history of prostate cancer, and being from certain ethnic backgrounds. It is thought that many genetic changes are involved in the development of prostate cancer. Some genetic changes have been discovered that can cause a large increase in prostate cancer risk and, occasionally, just one of these changes running through a family can be the cause of prostate cancer. Such changes are known to be very rare but thought to be more common in men who are diagnosed at a younger age (i.e. under 70 years) and men with a more aggressive disease.

More common genetic changes have been identified that can increase or decrease a man's risk of prostate cancer, each by a small amount. A "genetic profile" is the process of screening someone's DNA for many of these common changes and adding them all together to give an overall genetic risk score.

The study aims to look at how we can combine information of both rare and common genetic changes into a genetic test to be used in future clinical practice. We aim to recruit 1,000 men with prostate cancer, and 1,000 men closely related to someone with prostate cancer, at the Royal Marsden over a period of six years to undergo research testing.

Why have I been invited?

You are potentially eligible for the study. There are two groups of men we are inviting:

1. *Men who have had a diagnosis of prostate cancer*

AND

 (a) *who were diagnosed under the age of 70 OR*

 (b) *have advanced prostate cancer (and diagnosed at any age) OR*

 (c) *also have a close relative with prostate cancer.*

2. *Men who have a strong family history of prostate cancer but who have not had prostate cancer*

themselves. For the purposes of this study a family history of prostate cancer is defined as either:

(a) Having a first degree relative (father, brother or son) diagnosed with prostate cancer under the age of 70 years OR

(b) Having two relatives on the same side of the family diagnosed with prostate cancer, where one was diagnosed under the age of 70 OR

(c) Having three relatives on the same side of the family diagnosed with prostate cancer at any Age.

[They will take your DNA and compare it with others who also develop cancer. Their findings may show you if are more likely to develop cancer]

Of this criteria, 1(b) and (c) and 2(a), (b) and (c) applied to my own circumstances. I was therefore eligible to take part in the programme and attended the Royal Marsden for an interview and blood tests on the 1st June 2022.

At this meeting my family history was reviewed in detail and I was told that the analysis of the blood and genetic tests would take around six to nine months.

I was also asked if members of my family would be interested in participating in the ongoing studies. This would be my two sons, my two nephews (my sister had died from ovarian cancer) and my older living aunt who had experienced several forms of cancer, including ovarian cancer.

I was very willing and interested to take part in this research as any findings may go towards early diagnosis and treatment.

I was contacted on the 7th November 2002 with the first set of results:

The laboratory team have examined the DNA in your tumour sample, checking for spontaneously occurring genetic alterations in a number of genes associated with prostate cancer growth and **no alterations were identified.**

The laboratory team have also examined the DNA in your blood sample, checking for heritable high-risk genetic alterations in a number of genes associated with prostate cancer risk. **No high-risk genetic alterations were identified in these genes.**

On the 13th June 2023 I had a telephone follow-up conversation which outlined the entire procedure.

This was followed by a letter which detailed in layman's terms the two parts of the genetic testing that had been undertaken:

Part 1: We tested your DNA sample for mutations in known high-risk cancer genes that have been suggested to be involved in the development of prostate cancer. We did not find any known cancer-causing mutations in your sample. The list of genes that were tested can be found on the enclosed report.

Part 2: We analysed your polygenic risk score which estimates that using your genetic information alone your risk of developing prostate cancer by age 80 would be estimated to be 0.58 which suggests that you are at a lower than average risk of developing prostate cancer.

I was surprised at the outcome of the tests as I had been convinced that I had a genetically inherited prostate cancer from my father. This, however, was proven not to be so and the low reading that predicted my likelihood of getting the disease showed that I was just extremely unlucky.

To sum up: many thanks to the Royal Marsden for their thorough investigations into my family background. Both of my sons and one of my nephews are carrying on with continued testing.

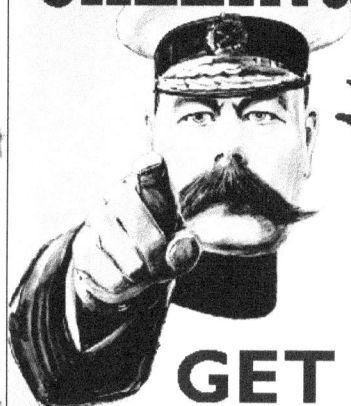

Chapter Twelve
PROSTATE CANCER: NOW THE MOST COMMON CANCER IN THE UK

Prostate cancer is now the most commonly diagnosed cancer, in the UK, with cases having risen by 25 percent in the past five years, NHS data has revealed.

Analysis by Prostate Cancer UK shows that prostate cancer has overtaken breast cancer. 55,033 men received a prostate cancer diagnosis. In 2023, while there were 47,526 breast cancer cases. This accelerated a trend from 2022, when 50,751 men were told they had prostate cancer while there were 48,531 breast cancer diagnoses.

The figures have put pressure increased pressure on ministers to overhaul the current "outdated" testing guidelines and implement the first national screening programme to save thousands of lives.

Experts said the "huge rise" in diagnoses was largely due to increased awareness. Celebrities, including Sir Stephen Fry, Bill Turnbull and Sir Chris Hoy have revealed their diagnoses. Although King Charles' type of cancer has not been revealed, it has been disclosed that he has received treatment for an enlarged prostate.

More men are living into their seventies and eighties, when the risk is highest, and diagnoses also soared after the pandemic because thousands of men missed out on tests during Covid lockdowns.

Despite it being the country's most common type of cancer, there is no routine screening programme for prostate cancer, unlike for breast, bowel and cervical cancer.

Under NHS guidelines, men over the age of 50 can ask their GP for a PSA test, even if they do not have symptoms.

Chapter Thirteen
OVARIAN CANCER: LINKED TO PROSTATE CANCER?

This year, 2025, it is predicted that approximately more than 55,000 men will be diagnosed with metastatic prostate cancer and nearly 7,500 women will be diagnosed with ovarian cancer. *(Cancer Research Statistics)*

Although it is not always known what causes cancer, there could be a family or genetic connection.

As many as one in four cases of ovarian cancer and one in 10 cases of metastatic prostate cancer show that it is caused by an inherited cancer syndrome.

Genetic testing (such as I, and my family, have had (and are still having) may be an option for those with a personal history or strong family connection to these cancer types.

If this is the case, your consultant will need to recommend referral to somewhere like The Royal Marsden Hospital.

Chapter Fourteen
ROYAL SURREY CANCER CENTRE

All of my diagnoses, treatments and follow-ups have taken place at St Luke's Cancer Centre in Guildford (part of the Royal Surrey County Hospital) which has just recently undergone a multi-million pound refurbishment which will now see it as one of Europe's leading surgical facilities. It has been renamed the Royal Surrey Cancer Centre. But for me it will always be the St Luke's Cancer Centre.

I am fortunate in that this centre of excellence is only two miles from my home.

The doors to its current home were first opened by Queen Elizabeth II and the former Duke of Edinburgh in 1997. Its history does, however, go back more than 60 years with the establishment of a cancer centre at the old St Luke's Centre in Warren

Road, Guildford (the one where my father received his treatment in 1990) and the first in the UK to introduce a Betatron electron therapy unit – the most advanced form of cancer treatment at the time.

The Royal Surrey Cancer Centre is now one of the country's major cancer centres, offering rapid diagnosis, advanced treatments and access to cutting-edge research to more than 8,000 patients each year. The Centre delivers more than 4,000 chemotherapy treatments, almost 3,500 sessions of radiotherapy and over 2,000 cancer surgeries annually.

Each prostate cancer patient receives individual assessment, analysis and diagnosis. A team of specialists, known as a multi-disciplinary team (MDT), will meet to discuss your cancer and recommend the most appropriate treatment. The MDT team includes surgeons, oncologists, radiologists, pathologists and specialist nurses.

Depending on individual circumstances, one or more of the following may be recommended:

Active Surveillance
Some people may not require any treatment and can be kept under active surveillance. This will

involve some or all of such things as regular PSA tests, MRI scans and biopsies. All carried out to ensure that any signs of progression are found as early as possible.

Prostatectomy

Radical prostatectomy is the surgical removal of the prostate gland. This treatment is an option for curing prostate cancer that has not spread beyond the prostate or has not spread very far.

Prostatectomies are performed using robots. Unlike traditional surgical methods, this avoids the trauma of an incision into the abdomen and organs being moved about. The machines allow the surgeons to use a control console to manoeuvre the robots' arms using a minimally invasive approach, known as keyhole surgery. Patients benefit from a shorter hospital stay, quicker recovery, reduced blood loss and less post-surgery discomfort.

The procedure, which is performed under general anaesthetic, takes around one and a half hours. Patients may, in some cases, be sent home the next day after being taught how to remove the catheter.]

Please read Tim's Story on page 93 for more details of this treatment

Brachytherapy

Brachytherapy is a form of radiotherapy where the radiation dose is delivered inside the prostate gland. It is delivered using a number of tiny radioactive seeds surgically implanted into the tumour. It is usually a day-case treatment and patients quickly return to their daily routines.

Brachytherapy may be used alone or in conjunction with hormone therapy or conventional radiotherapy, depending on the cancer.

Brachytherapy has the same high success rate as radical surgery but is believed to have fewer side-effects such as urinary leakage and impotence.

Please read Jeremy's Story on page 69 for more details of this treatment.

Radiotherapy

Radiotherapy involves using radiation to kill cancerous cells. It can be used to treat prostate cancer that has not spread very far from the prostate gland. It can also be used to slow the progression of prostate cancer that has spread and relieve the symptoms.

Please read David's story on page 107 for more details of this treatment

Hormone Therapy

Prostate cancer is fed by the male hormone, testosterone. This therapy blocks the production of testosterone and aims to stop the growth and spread of the cancer, in some cases shrinking it.

Hormone therapy is often recommended for patients with advanced prostate cancer and is initially given by an oral tablet, although some patients may also receive an injection that will be administered by a nurse or GP. This can be the main treatment or given in combination with one of the other treatments noted previously.

This is where I am at present but who knows what the future may bring.

Xofigo ®

Xofigo® is a treatment for patients with prostate cancer that has spread into the bones. Xofigo® can help relieve bone pain, slow the disease progression and reduce the likelihood of complications, such as bone fractures. It has been shown to improve life expectancy.

All of the this information has been taken from the Royal Surrey website:

royalsurrey.nhs.uk.

There is a wealth of information here, including videos and links to other sites.

From my own experience, I have a team of professionals who I am able to contact at any time. My main contacts, Claire and Sarah, have always been very helpful and responsive. I value and appreciate their dedication.

PERSONAL ACCOUNTS

The following pages contain personal accounts of family and friends who are have experienced, and are still experiencing the effects of, prostate cancer.

They show differences between GP assessments, diagnoses and treatments.

One sure thing is that if this killer disease is caught in time, the cancer can be treated and allows those affected to lead a normal life. With ongoing monitoring it gives those who are affected peace of mind and a positive future for themselves and their families.

I asked three men I know well to give me an insight into their diagnoses and treatments. I personally know of several more men who are also suffering and each one has a different tale to tell.

The three contributors are:

Jeremy, my younger son who lives in Cranleigh, just outside Guildford. He worked for Lloyds Bank for his entire working life and, now retired, devotes time to his family and volunteering at the Cranleigh Arts Centre where has organised their annual Cranleigh Book Festival for the past two years. He is married to Treena and they have one son, Fin, just coming up to 18 years old.

Tim, lives in Liverpool, but is a Hitchin man. He and I go way back, having worked together for many years together in the printing industry. Tim is a keen cyclist and cook, his speciality being bread and souffles. Married to Melanie, they have one daughter Alanah who got married to Jack last year. His company produced our "Pocket and Patch" koala charity book in 2002 – thank you Tim!

David, a Scot, who lives in Leicester. We got to know each other when, along with his wife, Catriona, they set up a very successful publishing business and I represented one of the printing firms that produced their books. At the time of his diagnosis and treatment David and Catriona lived in Bath.

The final account is by my wife, Margaret (M to everyone). It reveals how this cancer affects a deep and loving relationship – and how we try to overcome the ups and downs.

Jeremy's Story
A NORMAL CUP OF TEA

February 2022 – a normal day and a normal meeting for a normal cup of tea with my dad should have been just that – except it wasn't.

In fact, it was anything other than normal and, unknown to me at the time, destined to set me off on a journey I wasn't thinking of having.

Dad and M always set off to Spain at the end of February each year, for six or seven weeks to catch the end of the winter sun, and I can't remember anything ever getting in the way of that. We'd arranged a get-together at a local café for a catch-up before they set off: an hour to discuss how bad Spurs had been doing, the merits of Boris Johnson and whatever else came to mind. I thought I'd be saying farewell and only seeing them via Facetime until early April.

So, when my dad said that they were to fly out on the Monday and return just 10 days later, the question marks started flying. Of course, they made up some flimsy excuse about going to a residents' meeting, and getting to the truth had an element of teeth-pulling about it, but eventually they revealed that he'd been diagnosed with stage four prostate cancer and needed to be back in the UK for the start of his chemotherapy treatment.

Not a normal cup of tea.

I hoped it was a relief for him to share his diagnosis. Some things are meant to be kept from your adult children. I didn't think this was one of them.

I'm a matter-of-fact sort, bad news doesn't faze me, you just have to play the cards dealt to you and I saw this as nothing different, despite dad about to board the gloomy treadmill of numerous hospital visits and depressing chemotherapy. But there's no going back.

I'd had always had regular PSA tests as part of my annual workplace BUPA medical and scored an impressive 0.9 or thereabout every times. However, I was now retired from work and hadn't had my PSA checked for a couple of years. In the light of my dad's diagnosis we all felt it prudent for me to undertake an up-to-date test. Nothing to fear.

My local GPs surgery in Cranleigh is excellent – no waiting for a nurse's appointment, straight in for the taking of a bit of blood. Very painless, very routine and a telephone appointment booked for later in the week to give me the result.

My doctor phoned, as arranged, and that's when events started to take an unexpected turn. Having a single PSA test is, in itself, just an indicator of the moment. Having regular (annual being ideal) PSA tests give you a baseline on which future tests are hung and I cannot overstate the importance for anyone wondering if getting tested is worthwhile. Creating a trend is extremely important, as I was about to find out.

The doctor told me that my PSA score had risen to 3.5. As stand-alone, that could be interpreted as nothing to be concerned about and it could be expected for someone of my age. In fact, had that been my first ever test, it might have been shrugged off as normal. However, the jump from my established reading of 0.9 (albeit a couple of years previously) was a big one – a cause for at least one raised eyebrow and I was summoned to the surgery in order to have a finger poked up my arse.

So there I was, a couple of days later. As I pulled my trousers back up, the doctor was pleased to tell me that my prostate was as smooth as a peach and nothing like a walnut – why doctors always need to explain things with fruit and nut related references, I don't really understand, but there it was and I'd always preferred a peach to a walnut anyway.

I explained my route to her door: outlining my dad's situation, which led to a bit of chin-thumbing – never a good thing in a doctor's consulting room, but she was clear it would be in my interests to have an MRI scan, just to be sure. A belt and braces type of thing as, apparently, a PSA and a finger up the bum are not the final authority on a cancer-free prostate. Who'd have thought? I shrugged and agreed. Nothing to fear.

In fact, looking back, I'm pleased and grateful that she thought it wise to refer me at that point. If my dad had been afforded the same courtesy, perhaps things wouldn't have gone so wrong so quickly for him – certainly his GP would have sent me home and told me all was well. Another lesson for us all.

So, just a few days later – impressive how fast things can move – I arrived at the Stokes Centre for Urology at the Royal Surrey County Hospital in Guildford. I hate hospitals. All that smell of antiseptic and ill people is enough to make me feel unwell, but the reception area at the Stokes Centre was doing its best to shrug this off and as I waited among a number of men, twenty years my senior, I felt nicely calm and collected.

Prior to the scan, the staff needed to know that my bladder was working as it should be, so they asked me to do a flow test. This involves doing something that we all find difficult – peeing on demand. I hadn't known I'd be asked to do this and was grateful that I had consumed two cups of tea that morning, otherwise I'm not sure how long I might have been there. Other patients were being provided with copious amounts of water to help them along which, I thought, might take a few hours to work its way through. The test itself requires you to pee into some sort of apparatus which measures the evenness of your stream of piss (who'd have thought?) and afterwards, I was subjected to an ultrasound of my bladder to see how well I'd emptied – I passed with flying colours on both accounts. Good to know. Next time I play Monopoly perhaps I should buy the Water Works as a tribute to my fully functioning bladder.

I spent a good twenty minutes in the scanner – a lot of clicks and whirrs and other loud noises – before being booked a results appointment for just a few days later. This time it would be face-to-face. Nothing to worry about.

Results Day: A rather round, dour-looking consultant greeted me on my return, offered me a chair and set about loading the images taken earlier that week. He turned the monitor towards me, revealing what looked like an image of a bright, full moon, and began to point out what a good-looking prostate I appeared to have, if there can be such a thing – the James Dean or Elvis Presley of prostates, maybe. Nice and round – peach-like, just as my GP had told me, with no indication of anything sinister in the slightest, just as I thought it would be. Not a walnut in sight.

So, that was that. A couple of weeks of NHS time to get to the right result.

The consultant then began to ask me a few questions about what had brought me here, a bit like my GP had. I explained about the increase in my PSA reading and my family history, how my dad had recently been diagnosed with prostate cancer, my paternal grandfather had died from it, my mother had had breast cancer, aged 61, and one of my paternal aunt had died from ovarian cancer.

As I reeled off the list, I realised it sounded like a pretty interesting set, something worthy of applause, maybe, although the consultant didn't appear to share the same view. He sat thumbing his chin, then thumbing it a bit more as I finished telling him about my impressive family cancer-related CV.

"You know," he said. "An MRI scan isn't as sensitive as you might think." Now you tell me. "If there was a small issue, it would be unlikely to pick it up." It appeared my peach might be very slightly nutty after all.

"It's always best to catch these things early," he said. "I think you should have a biopsy, just to be on the safe side. A sort of belt and braces kind of thing," he said.

As I looked at him, I wondered just how many belts and pairs of braces a man with a healthy-looking prostate actually needed. A few, it seemed.

He told me it was a short and painless experience, delivered under local anaesthetic, before uttering the words that no man wants to hear...

"We go in between your ball-sack and your arse," he said. Words to chill an eskimo, but when you're in the hands of capable professionals, all you can do is nod and agree to come back for the humiliation. So that's what I did, nothing but thoughts of my ball-sack and arse filling my head. Nothing to worry about.

The problem was that my dad, having undergone this procedure, had told me all about his prostate biopsy and I was unable to think of anything else in the lead up to mine.

The appointment came through quickly and I was back at the Stokes Centre within a couple of weeks, which was now less than a couple of months since my unusual cup of tea.

The first thing I should say is that nothing can prepare you for this type of thing, the second is that the changing room where you put on one of those pathetically flimsy gowns, should have a box by the door, marked "DIGNITY", where you can leave all of yours for the following half hour.

So, once I had donned the gown (having completed another successful flow test), I was ushered into a small room where I felt a mild sense of panic as, for the size of the space, four people were gathered around one of those hospital beds. Four! I had no idea why. The consultant biopsy-taker was a good-humoured middle-aged woman, flanked by two young nurses. An older man stood to the side of the bed as, apparently, some sort of hand-holding chaperone. He introduced himself as Keith and assured me that the procedure was nothing to worry about and that he'd had it a few years back, although his had been under a general anaesthetic – so he hadn't really gone through what I was about to have, but I wasn't in the mood to argue the point.

With a weird sense of trepidation I lay back on the bed, wondering why there were so many people there, but afraid to ask as my legs were plonked into the accompanying stirrups before one of the nurses lifted my gown at the front, exposing everything I feared would be exposed, although I guess there's no making omelettes without breaking a few eggs.

At this point, I wondered what the purpose of the gown actually was, seeing as it now just covered my chest. I might as well have entered the room stark naked for all the good it was doing. I'm sure no-one would have batted an eyelid, but my mind was trying to ignore the drafty feeling further down. So, there I was – laying on my back, legs in the air with three women of varying ages staring right up my arse. The feeling of vulnerability and awkwardness couldn't have been worse.

Then it did get worse as one of the nurses decided it was time to tape up my scrotum and get it out of the way, so to speak, which seemed like a good idea as no-one wants a wrinkly old sack spoiling their view, do they? I wouldn't, and there was always the possibility of a stray needle. I also wondered if it was that particular nurse's sole function and how it would make that evening's dinner table conversation.

Next came the local anaesthetic. I looked at the needle – Fuck! – it was a big one, confirmed as my eyes nearly left my skull as she pushed it in. Twice. If you think having an injection at the dentist is painful, think again, and I felt every inch of it, and I felt myself squeezing Keith's hand.

Once numb, I prayed it would be time to get started – the sooner it began, the sooner it ended – but I'd forgotten that they needed to insert an ultrasound probe to make sure the biopsy needles were being delivered to the right place. So, yes, any remaining self-respect I felt I might have had evaporated in the room as the consultant lubed up then thrust a large, dildo-shaped implement up my arse. Lucky for me, the numbing had already taken hold and, by this time, I was past caring.

Now, the biopsy involves taking sixteen samples from right across the prostate gland by using a rotating device, pre-loaded with the needles, that are then positioned and shot quickly into the gland and then retracted with a sample of tissue. Prior to the procedure, I had been asked if they could take some additional samples to help with research, so it would be eighteen in my case – in for a penny and all that. Another two weren't going to add to my embarrassment.

So, legs up, numbed, ball-sack taped, probe inserted, perineum nicely prepped, off she went.

At first, the noise is a little unsettling, the crack of a sniper rifle adding some mirth to the proceedings. I imagined Bernie the Bolt loading a crossbow for the consultant and her taking aim from fifty yards away left a bit, right a bit etc., or that she'd come in dressed up in Lincoln Green; such are the images in your head to keep you from reality.

Stranger still, was the relaxed and informative conversation throughout; which revolved around the embarrassment of the whole thing and the process itself.

As the needles shot in and out, the consultant told me that the procedure is still sometimes done under general anaesthetic for some patients – or wimps, as I would have thought – due to things like a fear of needles, or something like having weak anal muscles so the probe won't stay put; going on to enlighten the room that, apparently, my anus was "quite the gripper", something to be proud of and I live in hope of finding a use for that information before I die.

I found myself counting the bangs from the biopsy machine, counting down in relief that it was over. I can honestly say I've never been so glad to get my scrotum untaped, my functionless gown off and my clothes back on, with a telephone appointment made for the end of that week to give me the results. Nothing to worry about.

The call came on time, the doctor confirming they'd taken eighteen samples – yes! yes!– and they'd been sent for analysis – yes! yes! – and that seventeen had been returned negative.

What? Seventeen? Not eighteen?

By some stroke of luck, depending on how you look at it, one of my samples showed a very low grade cancer, three millimetres long, Gleason score seven. Who'd have thought it? There are some things you are prepared for, others not quite so and, although the initial words were unexpected, I still felt relatively calm about the whole thing. I had cancer, apparently, but a very, very minor type, minuscule risk and prostate cancer is one of the most common types of cancer in men in the UK. Despite the diagnosis, I felt like a bit of cancer fraud, really.

The doctor was nicely reassuring; telling me that I shouldn't be worried and how it was key to catch these things early, but it was clear that I would need to consider what I did next.

Back I went to the Stokes Centre, which was, by now, becoming my second home, for a chat about what the results meant in reality.

A young doctor put me at my ease – all smiles and small-talk – and reiterated that it was by mere chance that I was sitting in front of her. It would never have been discovered had not each of my medical professionals done their bit – my GP in recognising the significance of a not unusual PSA test, and the MRI consultant for referring me for a biopsy because of my unusual family history, and I was thankful for it, although I still couldn't decide whether knowing I had some horror growing slowly between my ball-sack and arse was a good thing. I thought it probably was. She proceeded to tell me that, at this point for me, the disease is very slow-growing and that it could be at ten years, maybe longer, before it started to cause problems – but problems it would undoubtedly cause.

She then outlined my options, of which there were two. The first, and most obvious, was to do nothing, just wait until I actually needed something doing. They'd monitor my PSA more closely – every six months – make sure all was well, with maybe the occasional MRI scan. Known as *active surveillance*.

The second was something called *brachytherapy*; a treatment designed specifically for early, low-grade prostate cancer which involves implanting a quantity of tiny, radioactive seeds directly into the prostate to kill off the cancer. A form of targeted, internal radiotherapy without the side-effects of the traditional method of radiotherapy. I was told it would cure what I had. Appealing, but I wondered if that was really necessary at this stage.

Either way, I was happy to now be in a system that would look after me for the rest of my life. I opted for active surveillance and set a date for my next PSA test – November 2022.

The interim months were interesting. You might think you'd know what to do with even a small amount of cancer living inside you. But, until you get to do it, it's impossible to be sure. It was handy and comforting to have my dad to talk things through with and to have a laugh about it with. We shed tears of laughter over our shared biopsy experiences, cursed his GP many times and kept everything reassuringly normal. On the whole, I was very upbeat, with only the occasional foray into the worst-case scenario.

I returned to the nurse at my GP surgery for my next PSA test. I felt that nothing had changed for six months. Nothing to fear.

The Stokes Centre fielded the result calls, so when they rang a week later, I wasn't expecting anything unfortunate, which turned out to be a case of expectation not met, as the nurse revealed my latest PSA score had jumped all the way up to 10. Being in double figures for some things can be a cause for celebration – not, though, in this case.

"It's a bit high," said the nurse. No shit, I thought, wondering how on earth I could have gone from 3.5 to 10 in the space of a few months. "It could be that the cancer is more active," she said, not to reassure me, obviously.

Now my mind started to mumble in my ear about what was happening in my body. I thought about my dad and how such a delay had left him in a vulnerable position; I considered that I might have been wrong to opt for active surveillance and whether the cancer was trying to break out into other parts of my body. Plenty to worry about.

On the advice of the Stokes, I got re-tested the following week, just in case it was some sort of false reading. This time, the result came back at 6.3. A reduction, but still nearly double what it had been. I've never been one to worry about my own mortality, but, I guess that's the case until something comes along to remind you about it and I felt this knocking on my door. I looked at my wife, and then my son, and found myself hoping I'd be around to see him reach adulthood. Irrational thoughts, maybe, but that's where one's mind can wander.

Most difficulties in life are easily overcome by taking control of the situation and this, I felt, was no different.

I called the team at the Stokes and said I wanted to proceed with brachytherapy, rather than hang around. A cure is a cure, after all. The nurse I spoke to told me that she thought my decision was a good one and that they'd get me in for treatment at the next available opportunity. Again, I was pleased with the speed with which they made things happen, not the usual NHS horror story of waiting lists and missed opportunities. Far from it.

I was booked in for the procedure the following February, more or less, exactly a year since the unusual cup of tea and within three months of my own tests. In the interim, I was required to have a full ultrasound scan of my prostate to get its exact dimensions as the iodine-infused seeds had to be ordered from the USA. Yes, you've guessed it, it involved having a probe stuck up my arse again. Strange, the things you can get used to, and that was beginning to became a familiar phrase to my ears.

I did a bit of research and was comforted to learn that the Stokes Centre is the largest in Europe for performing the brachytherapy procedure and has a theatre used specifically for this purpose. On the day, I noted that there were patients there from right across the country, some having travelled hundreds of miles to be treated at my local hospital. Very reassuring.

Also reassuring was that this was to be done under general anaesthetic. Someone would undoubtedly be staring at my scrotum, but I wouldn't be awake to stare back.

Another flow test and ultrasound to check for adequate bladder emptying got the thumbs up. The procedure itself lasts about thirty minutes. Due to my relatively young age, something called space gel was added to the area between my prostate and my rectum to create a temporary space to protect the rectum from any leakage from the radioactive seeds which, rarely, can lead to secondary cancers which, seems to me, kind of defeats the object of the brachytherapy in the first place.

I awoke, none the wiser, feeling just like I had before I went in (once the catheter was removed, that is, OOF!).

I spoke to the surgeon who assured me that all had gone well and, after I had demonstrated my ability to pass water, I was allowed home. Home in time for lunch as if not much had happened – my kind of cancer treatment, for sure.

I was given a leaflet about the possible side effects of the treatment which included bladder discomfort, urine retention, changes in bowel habits and erectile problems. Thankfully, the only issue I had, which only lasted for a week or so, was that peeing was like squeezing water out of a balloon with a knot tied in the end. It took me a good few minutes to empty my bladder at the rate of a dripping tap and I had to get up a couple of times in the night, but I considered that a small price to pay.

I was also provided with a letter and a wallet-sized, laminated card to be produced if I had any third-party issues, specifically when going through security scanners at airports. Apparently, for the first two years following the implants, a very sensitive scanner might pick up some radioactivity from the seeds and no-one wants that in Departures.

I pictured myself being taken to one side by airport security, having to explain that my radioactive bollocks weren't, in fact, some sort of advanced micro-nuclear device and that I wasn't determined to set off on the plane and that Al-Qaeda hadn't recruited some middle-aged white guy from the Surrey Hills and filled his scrotum with super-enriched uranium. Anyway, I was grateful for the thought and, as it turned out, had no issues whenever I travelled, subsequently.

So, that was that. There ended my brief brush with prostate cancer and I felt I had been both lucky and unlucky at the same time.

Now I am on regular reviews with the Stokes Centre, which is basically a six-monthly PSA test, moving on to annual reviews after a couple of years, with associated phone calls to check that I'm okay. My PSA score is now back to normal.

As a by-product of my situation and my dad's treatment, The Royal Marsden Hospital got in touch to ask if I would help them with their genetic testing programme, specific to prostate cancer. I was obviously on their radar due to the information about my family history and the impressive list of cancers therein. I really couldn't blame them.

I had a single visit and consultation at the Marsden – a twenty minute chat with a research scientist which didn't yield any new information which was followed by them taking of a few phials of blood so they could establish if I was carrying any of the currently recognised genes associated with prostate cancer.

I was to be included in two projects, one to screen for four specific genes, the other to cast a wider net in their research into other potential indicators.

I was happy to help. Both for the greater good and also to learn if I might have passed anything down to my son.

The results came back negative. I don't appear to have any genetic predisposition to the disease which was both reassuring and discouraging, as I was left to ponder the fact that it was just a case of very bad luck that I had started to develop the disease. Case closed. Nothing to worry about.

When all is said and done, there are lessons that came from my experience which I want to pass on.

First, the importance of getting tested if you are over fifty, or if there is a history of prostate cancer in your family. Like I said earlier, establishing a PSA baseline over a number of years is essential to a healthy future.

Second, if your PSA hikes, don't be fobbed off by your GP. Insist on an MRI scan at least: it might just save your life.

Tim's Story

In 2013, when I was 50, my GP's surgery called me in for what they called a "Well Man's" health check. How enlightened, I thought.

It transpired to be a blood test for vitals, blood pressure check, my weight and a chat about my lifestyle choices. Ironic because as an active person who participated in sport at least six times a week, a home cook who prepares food from fresh and very rarely eats a ready meal, I found it odd to be given a lecture by someone that quite obviously didn't practice what they were preaching. Anyhow, I asked about my prostate as news articles at the time were heightening awareness of prostate cancer risks in men of all ages. I was told that they would not do a PSA blood test as I did not fall into the age bracket for testing and that the blood test threw up too many false positives.

As the years rolled on, I increasingly suffered some lower abdominal pain and regular visits to the GP concluded that I was suffering from a bi-lateral inguinal hernia. It was too small to operate on and therefore the best thing for me to do was work on my muscular core to help with the problem. I have always suffered from back issues and the thought of doing endless sit-ups was not an option, so yoga was the way to go.

Then in 2017, with increasing pain and not being able to lay on my left-hand side, I went back to the GP, outlined my symptoms and asked that something to be done. The decision was a hernia operation and sometime later I received the call to go for the pre-op and then an appointment for outpatients' surgery. Having fasted for well over twelve hours, as instructed, I stood naked as the day I was born in front of a female surgeon who asked me to point to where the pain was and, with marker pen in hand, she drew the most perfect arrow in one swoosh of the pen. I was told to wait there as she left the room. On her return, she was accompanied by another surgeon who asked me what my problems were and then with a prod and a poke said he could see no demonstrable evidence that my condition was hernia related and whilst he could perform the operation, he did not feel that it would resolve my problem, so he prescribed getting dressed, going home and having a good steak dinner. He, in turn, would refer me to a urologist.

Some weeks passed and the urology department at the Countess of Chester Hospital in Liverpool called me in for an appointment. I ran through the circumstances and symptoms that had led me to this point. A rectal examination showed no cause for concern, and a quick into pee in a bucket to measure my urinary flow showed a good flow and, as a precaution, a PSA blood test would be done. I walked away without worrying about anything.

During this period, Melanie and I decided to splash a little cash and have the en-suite refurbished and while we were at the local tile wholesaler chatting through options of some very expensive floor-to-ceiling porcelain tiles the phone rang – an unknown number – it could be work, so. I politely excused myself and took the call. It was the hospital, my blood test had come back and both my PSA and cholesterol were through the roof. They wanted to re-test as they were not certain that there had been a laboratory error but, if not, it was highly likely to be cancer.

Nothing ever prepares you for that word, but at the mention of it your world just stops. I hung up, dazed and stunned, returned to Melanie and the salesman but my interest in tiles, whether they be porcelain or anything else, had disappeared. Melanie could see something was up and I am sure the salesman knew too. I couldn't get out of there quickly enough. Melanie and I sat in the car as I told her about my conversation as best as I could recollect it. Then we waited for the recall appointment to be re-tested.

In a matter of weeks, bloods were taken and then I had a follow-up appointment with another urologist. With very little preamble he told me I had cancer. I broke down in tears and whatever he said just didn't register. Thank heavens for Melanie, as the rock she is, did all the listening for me.

My PSA was 25 and my Gleason score was 7 (3+4). It turns out understanding whether it is 3+4 or 4+3 is very important – who knows that? They would need to perform a prostate biopsy to ascertain the extent of the disease – and the less said about that the better. It was one of the most unpleasant experiences of my life. Afterwards, they said I might pee a little blood, but it was nothing to worry about. Two days later, a tennis chum decided to take a select few of us for a birthday treat to go and watch Tranmere Rovers play Stevenage Town. Before moving North to Liverpool, I was a follower of Hitchin Town and the opportunity to watch Tranmere Rovers get one over on of Hitchin's old adversaries could not be turned down.

Anyhow, at half time, the need to visit the toilet was all-consuming and standing at the urinal shoulder-to-shoulder with others, the river ran red and the horror on the other men's faces was a picture to behold.

The weeks that passed just dragged by and I had to go about my working life as best I could. Being a salesman, I couldn't let it affect my outward persona, but at times it was tough. One of the most difficult meetings during this period was with a client in Bangor and, rather than cancel the meeting because her child minder had called in sick, she had to bring her little girl along. I sat there discussing business and it suddenly dawned on me that I might never get to see my daughter have children or experience grandchildren. At the end of the appointment and shortly after we parted, I found myself sitting in my car welling up.

The results were in (or at least at the hospital) and they were sent to what is known as an MDT (multi-disciplinary team (a collective of specialists in their field to decide what the best course of action was for my case. It was now a waiting game as they only met on a weekly basis and reviewed as many cases as possible in the limited time available to them before getting on with their house duties.

Days turned into weeks, weeks into months. It was now two months since my first diagnosis and my state of mind was anxious, to say the least, and during this time I had undergone MRI and CT scans to determine further the extent of the disease and whether there was any metastatic spread of the cancer.

The MDT met and I was given an appointment to have a joint discussion with both a surgical urologist and a radiologist on Friday the 23rd December 2017. We visited the local NHS cancer hospital at Clatterbridge to meet with the two specialists but only one, Mr Manal Kumar, was in attendance. After a short period of time, he rang the radiologist's secretary to try and find out where the other consultant, was, only to be told that as it was as good as Christmas Eve he'd decided to take the day off to go Christmas shopping and we were advised that he would write to us in the new year to rearrange.

Melanie and I are fortunate enough to have private health cover, so I immediately rang our provider to ask whether they would cover the consultation – "yes" was the answer.

We then rang the secretary back to ask when was the earliest the consultant could see us under private medical cover – Wednesday the 27th December was the response. We made the appointment and set about hearing what Mr Kumar had to say. It was the MDT's belief that, given my age, my health and my disease with no metastatic spread, the best option was to undergo a laparoscopic radical robotic prostatectomy.

The operation could be performed at the local NHS Arrowe Park Hospital where they had one of the few machines in the North West of England. The procedure would be under general anaesthetic and performed whilst I was inverted which involved tilting me head-down at a 45-degree angle to create space and optimise access for the robotic arms during the procedure This positioning helps the surgeon perform the delicate surgical steps involved in removing the prostate, while utilising the robotic arms system's precision and dexterity..

The operation consisted of six insertions and would be to remove the prostate, lymph nodes, seminal glands and any other affected parts. One downside to this procedure, he stated, was that I would never be able to father children afterwards and also that erections may not be as strong as previously. The upside for opting for this would be that if any cancerous cells were missed then targeted beam radiotherapy could be used. Opting for the latter first would rule out any laparoscopic radical robotic prostatecomy as they would not be able to operate due to the scar tissue. It was a no-brainer as far as we were concerned. It was Mr Kumar who would do this work, but we had to tick the NHS box and see the radiologist for him to explain his procedure.

Nine months earlier, Melanie and I had committed to rent a house in which to spend Christmas in our favourite part of Provence in France. That was now a non-starter; instead it would be a festive break at home and we resigned ourselves to a quiet one with just the two of us and whatever we could pick up at the supermarket for food – we would get by.

My sister-in-law, Joy, and her husband, Simon, would not have it. They insisted that we must spend Christmas with them in Manchester and what a welcome relief that turned out to be; much food, much wine and great company – a true tonic to help blow away the dark clouds that hung over us.

Following the consultation with the radiologist, we duly set about telling Mr Kumar that my preferred option was his recommendation and he set the wheels in motion. However, he needed to go away for a couple of weeks but gave me his email address in case I needed to contact him and he assured me he would respond as soon as he got a chance.

The date was set for the operation to take place on Saturday the 20th January 2018 but on the Friday we received a call from Mr Kumar to say that he could not perform the operation as Arrowe Park had cancelled all procedures deemed non-essential; they were in the midst of a winter flu outbreak and all beds were full. We then spent the coming days and weeks trying to get all the pieces of the jigsaw to fit – Mr Kumar could get the theatre staff, but then couldn't get the theatre, and then he couldn't get a bed, and so on and on it went. It was beginning to get me down, so Melanie booked us a weekend away in the Lake District to get our minds off the whole thing. We finally managed to get an agreement that the big day would be Saturday the 3rd February 2018 and with all that had gone before, I was nervous that it might fall through again.

We arrived at the hospital before the wards were even open to the public and a nurse let us in to sit in the waiting room. Mr Kumar came to see us and said that they still couldn't get a bed on a ward, but: "Don't worry, we are doing this." I got changed, told Melanie I loved her and was wheeled down to theatre where I was introduced to the team that would assist Mr Kumar and given a guided tour of the room. It was like something out of a sc-fi film – a very large room with a very large piece of equipment with bionic arms protruding and, in a corner a booth, where Mr Kumar controlled the beast and performed the operation.

I got onto the bed, counted backwards from 100 and got, from what I remember, to 90. Six hours later, I opened my eyes and asked when I would be having the operation only to be told, "It's all done and you're in ITU for recovery as there still aren't any beds available."

Once on the ward, I was so happy to see Melanie and our daughter, Alanah.

Mr Kumar did his rounds and came to see me. He proclaimed that, from his standpoint, the operation had been a success: he had removed the prostate, lymph nodes and seminal gland, as previously discussed, and whilst there had noticed that the disease had escaped the capsule, so he had therefore decided to remove some surrounding tissue. This had involved cutting through some nerves, but he was confident that they would rejoin and he reiterated that erections would not be as strong or as long as I had probably become accustomed to – a small price to pay, I thought.

I was out of the door on Monday morning and on my way home, having been told to keep mobile and reminded to work on my pelvic floor as I still had a catheter in but it would be removed a week later.

Daily walks around the block ensued, along with nightly self-injecting of something to help me recover. After a week, I went back to the walk-in clinic to check whether I could empty my bladder and, if so, the catheter would be removed – and it was – Thank Heavens! Walking around with a bag filled with urine is not, and never will be, a fashion accessory. They tell you before the operation to work on your pelvic floor as, with no prostate, there is no stopper and it is essential in staying dry.

Life quickly got back to normal and the wearing of incontinence pants for a short period of time was essential as, every so often, I'd get a surge and a resultant wet spot, often caused by the consumption of a little bit too much alcohol!

Post operation, I started off with quarterly PSA checks and these were anxious times, the tension palpable – did he get it all, will it come back? After twelve months, these turned into six monthly tests and checks. I was still tense in the times building up to them. Then on to an annual test when my PSA was/is non-existent with a reading of 0.0006 (undetectable). Mr Kumar says there is no need to keep going for a check-up as he is certain that there is no chance of any recurrence of the disease, but there is something reassuring to be told that your PSA is undetectable and, beside which, it's always good to catch up with Mr Kumar.

The six keyhole scars from the surgery have all but disappeared and perhaps the only thing that has really changed is the "salesman's bladder" – the ability to drive long distances and not have to stop for a pee – as now, when the urge comes, it is all-consuming. Other than that, life is as normal as it can be. I still play competitive tennis twice a week and cycle upwards of 60 miles a week, depending on the weather.

I wake every day and tell my darling Melanie that I love her as I would never have got through everything without her support and remind myself to be thankful as what I had to go through has been a walk in the park compared to her experience.

Melanie was diagnosed with Stage 4 breast cancer during lock-down in 2020. She is having to endure seemingly endless rounds of chemotherapy with all its ups and downs and in addition to the side effects that she is having to suffer just trying to keep this monstrous disease at bay.

David's Story
A JOURNEY
THROUGH
DIAGNOSIS AND
TREATMENT

In the autumn of 2016, it felt like the world had tilted slightly off its axis. I was 65, a retired publisher living a quiet life in Bath, Somerset. My days were filled with simple pleasures generally revolving around food and wine. Life was predictable, comfortable and enjoyable. But that September, a routine visit to Dr Howse at my local medical centre changed everything.

It started with a blood test, one of those annual check-ups I'd grown accustomed to. I didn't think much of it: blood draws, cholesterol monitoring, and the usual battery of tests that were just part of ageing. A week later, Dr Howse called me back to her surgery. Her tone was calm, but carried a weight I hadn't heard before. "Your PSA level is elevated," she said, her eyes steady, but kind. "It's at 8.9, which is higher than we'd like to see for someone of your age. In March it was 5.6, so that's quite a jump to 8.9". PSA (Prostate-Specific Antigen) was a term I was vaguely aware of; I knew it had something to do with prostate health, but there my knowledge ended. I nodded at Dr Howse, unsure of what this latest reading meant, but sensed a rising panic in me at this news.

Dr Howse leaned forward, her hands clasped on her desk. "It doesn't necessarily mean cancer," she said, anticipating my unspoken fear. "But we need to take a closer look. I'd like to examine your prostate, and, depending on what I find, we'll decide on the next steps." I agreed, although my stomach churned with unease. The exam was quick, but uncomfortable: a digital rectal exam, or DRE, as she called it. Her expression didn't betray much, but when she finished, she sat back and said: "Your prostate is a bit enlarged and there's a small area that's firmer than I'd like. I'm recommending you see a urologist for further tests."

That lunchtime, I sat at the kitchen table, a half-eaten sandwich in front of me as I stared at the scrap of paper where I'd scribbled terms like "PSA", "prostate", and "urologist". My wife, Catriona, noticed my distraction. "What's going on, David?" she asked, her voice soft, but insistent. I told her about my appointment and what Dr Howse had said. Her hand reached for mine, squeezing gently. "We'll figure this out together," she said. That night, sleep eluded me. The word "cancer" loomed like a shadow.

The urologist, Dr Patel, was a brisk, but empathetic man in his late forties, with a reassuring smile and a knack for explaining complex medical terms in plain language. At our first appointment, he reviewed my PSA results and performed another DRE. "The prostate does feel enlarged," he confirmed, "and the firmness could indicate something we need to investigate further. I'll recommend a biopsy to get a clearer picture." A biopsy. The word felt like a punch. I nodded, trying to keep my composure, while Catriona asked questions I hadn't thought of: What would the procedure involve? How soon could we get results? Dr Patel explained that the biopsy would involve taking small samples of prostate tissue using a needle guided by ultrasound. It would be done under local anaesthesia, and the results would take about a week to come through.

The biopsy was scheduled for early November. The days leading up to it were a blur of anxiety and distraction. It's hard to stop your mind racing ahead into the unknown once the word "cancer" has been mentioned. I tried to stay busy: mowing the lawn, fixing a squeaky door, anything to keep my mind off the what-ifs. Catriona was my rock, researching prostate conditions online and reassuring me that an elevated PSA could be caused by benign conditions like prostatitis or benign prostatic hyperplasia (BPH). We were getting good at this medical terminology thing. But the dread and gloom of prostate cancer hung over us, unspoken and ever-present.

The biopsy itself was uncomfortable but bearable. Lying on my side in a sterile room, I focused on the hum of the ultrasound machine as Dr Patel worked. "You're doing great, David," he said, his voice calm and steady. Afterwards, I felt a mix of relief and dread: relief that the procedure was over, dread for the results. The wait was agonising. I found myself checking my phone obsessively, even though I knew the results wouldn't come by text. Catriona suggested we go for longer walks to clear our heads, and those moments, with the crisp autumn air and the crunching of leaves underfoot, were small reprieves.

When the call finally came, it was Dr Patel himself. "David, the biopsy results are in," he said. "You do have prostate cancer, but it's early-stage, Gleason score 4+3. This is a low-grade cancer, which is good news; it's slow-growing and very treatable." My heart sank at "cancer", but lifted slightly at "treatable". Catriona was beside me, holding my hand, as we listened to Dr Patel on speakerphone. He explained my three options: active surveillance, surgery, or radiotherapy.

Active surveillance meant monitoring the cancer without any immediate treatment. But the idea of living with cancer, even a slow-growing one, made me uneasy. I knew I'd be thinking about it all the time, wondering what it was up to. No.

Surgery would entail a radical prostatectomy: an operation to remove the prostate gland, seminal vesicles, and, if necessary, any nearby lymph nodes. Apparently, this kind of surgery is a common treatment for prostate cancer, especially when the cancer is localised, like mine was. The goal is to remove all cancerous tissue, but the procedure carries risks, such as, incontinence and erectile dysfunction, which gave me pause for thought. As it happened, surgery wasn't an option for me anyway, because of a combination of factors; weak lungs from childhood asthma; the fact that I was a fat bastard with a BMI of 34 who also had hypertension and high cholesterol; and on top all that, a mouth too small to fit an intubation tube in, should any complications arise during the surgery.

Radiotherapy, Dr Patel explained, would target the cancer with minimal invasiveness, shrinking the prostate and eliminating the cancerous cells over several sessions.

After a long discussion with Catriona and a second opinion from the postman, I chose radiotherapy. Dr Patel referred me to a radiation oncologist, Dr Nguyen, who specialised in External Beam Radiation Therapy (EBRT). At our first meeting,. Dr Nguyen was meticulous, walking me through the process with diagrams and statistics. "We'll use twenty-one sessions of intensity-modulated radiation therapy (IMRT)," she said. "It's precise, targeting the prostate while minimising damage to surrounding tissues. You'll come in five days a week for about four weeks." She warned me about potential side effects (fatigue, urinary irritation, and possible bowel changes), but assured me they were usually temporary.

Prior to the radiation, on the 15th December 2016, I was given hormone treatment: Bicalutimide 50mgs to be taken once daily for two weeks total. The first radiation session was planned for mid-March 2017. The radiation centre in Bath, at the time of my treatment, was a modern facility with a calming atmosphere, soft music playing in the waiting room and staff who greeted me by my first name. Before starting the course of radiation, I underwent a planning session called a simulation, where technicians used a CT scan to map my prostate and create a customised treatment plan. They tattooed tiny dots on my pelvis to ensure precise alignment for each session. Lying on the treatment table, I felt like an astronaut preparing for launch, the machine humming and clicking as it positioned itself.

Each session was quick (not more than 15 minutes) and the daily routine became a strange rhythm in my life. I'd drive to the centre with Catriona, check in, change into a gown, and lie on the table while the linear accelerator delivered invisible beams of radiation. The technicians were kind, often chatting about the weather or local sports to put me at ease. Catriona came with me every morning. Getting the earliest appointment each day was a bonus, as it got the whole thing out of the way and meant we could plan a least an afternoon doing something, if we wanted to. Another bonus was the short drive from our house to the centre. Some patients travelled a long distance each day, which can only have added to their stress levels. Catriona was a steady and calming presence and it would have been a hell of a lot more stressful if I had been on my own.

At first I didn't notice any difference to how I felt, but the side effects crept in at around week two. Fatigue was the worst, a bone-deep tiredness that made even a short walk feel like a marathon. I started napping in the afternoons, something I'd never done before. Urinary irritation came next: frequent trips to the loo, and a burning sensation that made me wince. Dr Nguyen prescribed medication to ease the symptoms, and Catriona stocked the fridge with cranberry juice, which she swore would help. The bowel changes were milder, mostly occasional discomfort, but manageable. One strange and not unpleasant effect of the cancer treatment was my sudden love of cider. The Malbec remained untouched and neglected in the wine rack as Catriona and I scoured the Somerset countryside for cider producers. Neither of us could quite believe it. Through it all, I kept some notes, jotting down how I felt each day, partly to track my progress, partly the surreal experience of being "a cancer patient".

By the twenty-first session, just before Easter, I felt like a veteran of the radiation table. The final session was anticlimactic: no bells or fanfare, just a handshake from the technician and a "Well done, David!" from Dr Nguyen. She scheduled a follow-up PSA test for three months later and warned me that the radiation's side effects might well continue for some weeks. Driving home, I felt a mixture of relief and uncertainty. The treatment was over, but the journey wasn't.

The months that followed were a slow return to normal. The fatigue gradually subsided, and the urinary symptoms eased. My first post-treatment PSA test, in the summer of 2017, showed a level of 1.2ng/mL: a dramatic drop. Dr Patel called it excellent news, confirming that the radiation had done its job. Follow-up scans showed the prostate had shrunk significantly, and the cancer appeared to be in remission. The word "remission" felt like a gift, but I knew it came with caveats: regular check-ups, ongoing PSA tests, and the ever-present possibility of recurrence.

Looking back, the experience reshaped me in ways I hadn't expected. I'd always been a planner, someone who liked control, but cancer taught me how to live with uncertainty. It deepened my gratitude for Catriona, whose quiet strength carried us both through the darkest moments. It made me cherish the small things: the smell of coffee in the morning, leisurely walks through fields and woods, a nice glass of Malbec (the cider got kicked to the kerb as soon as I returned to "normal")....

So, in 2016, a raised PSA level was a wake-up call, a jolt that forced me to confront my mortality. The twenty-one sessions of radiotherapy were a challenge, but they were also a bridge to hope, a reminder that even in the face of fear, there's a path forward. Today, as I sit in my garden, watching the first buds of spring 2025 emerge, I'm grateful for all the doctors, the technology, and the love that carried me through. Life isn't perfect, but it's mine, and I'm still here to live it.

M's Story
HAVE YOU TAKEN YOUR TABLETS?

Our mantra for the day is: "have you taken your tablets?" The dining table now always has a strip of tabbies lurking on it and I mostly try to remind H to swallow one – don't chew it – he says they are vile to taste. You would think it's easy to remember, but we often digress into the day's activities and, oops, the moment is gone. Tabby not taken – remembered hours later.

Mindful of the future, Harry and I had often talked about if either or both of us were wiped out in a car or plane crash and had done our wills, leaving our property and hundreds of books accordingly – but it had always had a bit of the surreal feel about it. Not once had we thought of terminal illness and, do you know, I still don't, as I don't feel it applies to "us". That is what happens to "other people."

When my father-in-law died in 1990, I was hardly aware of prostate cancer. A few years later I had to spend two nights at the Royal Surrey County Hospital in a mixed ward, surrounded by elderly men, who had "prostate problems" and had received "treatment". Obviously, nothing we needed to worry or think about, just the "old man's disease" – we would never be old, would we?

When Harry started talking about getting his prostate checked, it didn't really register on my radar – yeah, whatever – you get the picture – just another bit of routine, like women's breast scans or cervical smear tests. I have never been the sort of person who dreads these, just go in, get your kit off and put up with the breast squeezing or cold speculum inside.

However, it all started to change when we were in Spain in October 2021 and H was talking seriously about pains in his groin. Typically, he didn't make any fuss, just saying: "I think I will get it checked out," and we moved on to talk out what was for lunch – probably chicken wings from Mercadona (our local Spanish supermarket) with home-made chips and salad (we like our food). I still didn't really think that much about it. A visit to the GP in

November seemed to allay any fears but they decided to do a PSA test.

Time went on and we were into January 2022 and, suddenly, off he was for a scan – the new doctor had recognised the possible implications of Harry's PSA reading which, combined with his father dying of prostate cancer and his sister of ovarian cancer, he realised what it might mean for this 77 year old man. This GP wasn't H's usual one – thank Christ – as he might be dead by now.

It suddenly became real and off we went: every week for a different scan – me dropping H off at various locations at the RSCH – luckily we live within two miles of the hospital – waiting in the car park (some hope!), or more likely the nearby Tesco, waiting for a call. I always took my phone so I could read my latest book (I am an avid reader) but, do you know, I don't think I ever recall reading a page. I was always "on edge" waiting and worrying. I could flip 20 pages and not remember what happened. Worse was to come when I had to drop H off and go home – how to fill those vacant hours? I had bought a new jigsaw puzzle of my beloved koalas (since 2022 we have donated hundreds of dollars to various Australian koala charities through sales of a book we published to boost their funds) but it was difficult to concentrate. Even though they were "just scans" it didn't stop the worrying. H always tells me not to worry; "it won't help, just do something nice for lunch – fish (cod or sole) or maybe one of your pies (Thai or Balti chicken)". H likes his food and I like cooking.

After the scans – a biopsy – I don't think I knew what that was (I do now – just read Jeremy's story). I do, however vividly recall collecting H afterwards, it was a desperately cold early winter evening and when, as you do, I enquired how it went, all he said was: "It wasn't too bad" and proceeded to tell me that one of the staff had been very interested in his koala badge (to go with our charity book). I took it at face value but, what a typically Harry-ish reaction (unbelievably painful, but just "OK"). I wish I had been more understanding and sympathetic, but that is not something my family does – keep smiling through and all that...

I had a cataract operation last year and after bringing me home, as soon as we stepped inside, H said: "any chance of a cuppa?" That's our sort of take on life: we may be bandaged and bleeding but life goes one, especially with a cuppa and a biscuit!

The day of the result of the biopsy and scans was a bit of an anti-climax – we knew what was coming – and I am not sure how I really felt and I can't ever remember us talking about it. However, I just wanted my beloved H to be well but knew in my heart, it would never be so. We just went home and had toast and marmite (lots of butter) – our "go-to" food. We wondered what would be next.

Chemo was next. "Let's not tell anyone," we decided. Five weeks at our house in Spain were already booked but that wasn't now possible. We could just about do 10 days. "We'll tell the family we are just going for a short trip as we need to go for the AGM of the residents' association". I knew Jeremy would never fall for that one – and as we sat in Roker's coffee shop (a farm shop just outside Guildford) he "grilled" us as to why we were not going for our usual five weeks. Eventually, H caved in and said: "I've got prostate cancer and will start chemo in just over two weeks". I had the pack of tissues at the ready: we all needed them that day.

So, off we went to Spain and, wow, did we make those ten days seem like five weeks! We didn't really talk about the future, just lived for the day: walks along the beach at La Mata and a cup of coffee, and lunches out. Although it was early in the year when the weather can be unpredictable, the sun shone every day (of course it did).

Chemo was the great unknown: what happened, how do you feel afterwards and, of course, what next? The first session was the first step. I usually went to Pilates on the day of the first session, so decided to forego that in case I was needed. I wasn't of course, and just festered at home. H settled in and sent me pictures of coffee and biscuits, followed by soup and sandwiches being delivered as he was being "chemoed". He was being waited on hand and foot, just as if he was at home! – albeit with a cannula in his arm for two hours. Me, I was looking at the Joey Koala jigsaw with a cooling cup of tea and thinking goodness knows what. I have never known a jigsaw puzzle take so long and have such soggy pieces through my tears – I cry very quickly and copiously as my family will tell you.

It became a standing joke between us that H would make sure not to leave the Chemo Ward until he had had his soup, sandwich, banana and piece of cake; the treatment certainly didn't affect his appetite. However, no lunchtime kitchen duty for me on those days!

Post-chemo didn't seem to be too bad, apart from having to give H an injection after the treatment. I had never done anything like this in my life, so to say it was daunting is an understatement. But, as with anything, one gets used to it and it quickly becomes the norm – what else might we have to become used to was a bit of a worry. But we took it in our stride.

H made light work of the chemo; where others lost weight and their hair, H just lost his hair – everywhere! H is the most phlegmatic of men and always says "we are where we are". It's a good philosophy to have – I wish I had it, as I often think: "If only that damned doctor had acted in 2020..." H wouldn't have had to endure chemo and all the other devastating drugs, etc.

Chemo has had its effects: hair loss, nail abnormalities, toe tinglies (neuropathy). The most dramatic effect, however, has been through the hormone treatment. This treatment suppresses his testosterone which feeds the cancer. For a very virile, healthy man this has been devastating for both of us. Additionally, the drugs cause weight gain which, for a man such as H, who has always been proud of his physique, has been life-changing.

H jokes about changing into a woman, which is very topical at present, but behind every joke there is an element of sadness – and pink has never been his favourite colour!

As a natural part of life, I am often the buffer between other people and H: "How is H?" "How is he really?" "What is the treatment doing to him?" I have to try and be honest but keep Harry's privacy. Neither he nor I want everyone to know what we know – of our low times. I look back on the change it has made to my own life; and thinking purely selfishly, it is huge. H and I have always been close and loving but the hormone treatment has taken away the physical element. One might think a couple in their seventies don't need this, but they would be wrong. But H and I make the best of it. There's no other way.

I don't always give H the support he deserves and I regret this. Why? I just don't know, perhaps he is just too accepting and I am just too resentful of the situation he is in. Whatever, I am grateful for every day we have and hope we have many more. We still belly-laugh over silly things, curse over Tottenham losing – again. I still cry at nothing and H is still here (thank God!) and taking the tablets, of course.